DR. SEBI ALKALINE DIET FOR CANCER: 5 BO(

Transform your health with potent alkaline diets and recipes to combat cancer and revitalize your body naturally

John Ernesto

Table of Contents

COPYRIGHT © 2023

BOOK 1

Understanding the Alkaline Diet and its Impact on Cancer

Introduction to the Alkaline Diet: Principles and Benefits

The alkaline diet is a dietary approach that emphasizes the consumption of alkaline-forming foods to maintain optimal pH levels in the body. Proponents of this diet believe that by consuming alkaline foods, such as fruits, vegetables, nuts, and seeds, and minimizing the intake of acidic foods, such as meat, dairy, and processed foods, one can achieve a more alkaline pH balance in the body, which is purported to offer various health benefits, including cancer prevention and treatment.

The fundamental principle behind the alkaline diet is based on the concept of pH balance. The pH scale measures the acidity or alkalinity of a substance and ranges from 0 to 14, with 7 being neutral. A pH below 7 is considered acidic, while a pH above 7 is alkaline. The human body tightly regulates its pH levels within a narrow range, primarily through the kidneys and lungs. However, proponents of the alkaline diet argue that modern diets high in acidic foods can disrupt this balance, leading to health problems, including cancer.

Advocates of the alkaline diet claim that maintaining a slightly alkaline pH balance in the body can help prevent cancer by creating an environment that is unfavorable for cancer cell growth and proliferation. Additionally, they suggest that following an alkaline diet can support conventional cancer treatments, such as chemotherapy and radiation therapy, by reducing side effects and enhancing their effectiveness.

How pH Balance Affects Cancer Growth and Progression

The relationship between pH balance and cancer growth and progression is a complex and multifaceted topic that has been the subject of extensive research and debate. While it is well-established that cancer cells can thrive in acidic environments, the role of pH balance in cancer development and progression is not fully understood.

Cancer cells exhibit a unique metabolic phenotype known as the Warburg effect, which involves a shift from oxidative phosphorylation to aerobic glycolysis, even in the presence of oxygen. This metabolic adaptation allows cancer cells to generate energy more efficiently and sustain rapid proliferation. Importantly, the acidic byproducts of glycolysis, such as lactic acid, contribute to the acidic microenvironment surrounding tumors, which can promote cancer cell survival, invasion, and metastasis.

In addition to the Warburg effect, the acidic tumor microenvironment also plays a role in modulating immune responses and promoting tumor angiogenesis (the formation of new blood vessels to support tumor growth). Acidic conditions can impair the function of immune cells, such as T cells and natural killer cells, thereby facilitating immune evasion by cancer cells. Furthermore, acidic pH levels can stimulate the production of angiogenic factors, such as vascular endothelial growth factor (VEGF), which promote the growth of blood vessels into the tumor, providing nutrients and oxygen essential for tumor growth and metastasis.

Given the critical role of pH balance in cancer biology, there is growing interest in targeting the acidic tumor microenvironment as a therapeutic strategy. Preclinical studies have demonstrated that buffering the acidity of the tumor microenvironment can inhibit cancer cell proliferation, enhance the efficacy of chemotherapy and immunotherapy, and reduce metastatic potential. However, translating these findings into effective clinical interventions remains a challenge, and further research is needed to develop safe and targeted approaches for modulating pH balance in cancer patients.

Scientific Evidence Supporting the Alkaline Diet's Role in Cancer Prevention and Treatment

The scientific evidence supporting the role of the alkaline diet in cancer prevention and treatment is limited and inconclusive. While some studies have suggested a potential link between dietary acid load and cancer risk, the overall evidence is mixed, and the mechanisms underlying any observed associations remain poorly understood.

A systematic review and meta-analysis published in the Journal of Environmental and Public Health in 2012 evaluated the association between dietary acid load and cancer risk. The analysis included 41 studies with a total of over 1.4 million participants and found a modest positive association between higher dietary acid load and overall cancer risk. However, the authors noted significant heterogeneity between studies and emphasized the need for further research to elucidate the biological mechanisms underlying this association.

In terms of cancer treatment, there is limited clinical evidence to support the efficacy of the alkaline diet as a standalone therapy or adjunctive treatment for cancer patients. While some small-scale studies and case reports have reported anecdotal benefits of adopting an alkaline diet in conjunction with conventional cancer treatments, such as improved quality of life and symptom management, the overall quality of evidence is low, and more rigorous research is needed to validate these findings.

One of the challenges in studying the alkaline diet's impact on cancer outcomes is the lack of standardized dietary interventions and outcome measures across studies. Additionally, dietary adherence and compliance can be difficult to assess and may vary widely among participants, further complicating the interpretation of study results.

Overall, while the alkaline diet may offer potential health benefits, including cancer prevention and treatment, the current scientific evidence is limited and inconclusive. Further research, including well-designed clinical trials with larger sample sizes and longer follow-up periods, is needed to elucidate the role of dietary pH balance in cancer biology and determine the efficacy of the alkaline diet as a therapeutic approach for cancer patients. In the meantime, individuals should consult with healthcare professionals before making significant dietary changes, especially if they have been diagnosed with cancer or are undergoing cancer treatment.

Key Principles of Dr. Sebi's Alkaline Diet Approach to Cancer

Dr. Sebi's alkaline diet approach to cancer is based on the belief that maintaining an alkaline environment in the body can support overall health and help prevent and manage various diseases, including cancer. Dr. Sebi, whose real name was Alfredo Darrington Bowman, was a self-proclaimed healer and herbalist who promoted a plant-based, alkaline-rich diet as a means of achieving optimal health and wellness. While his methods and claims have been controversial and subject to criticism, they have also garnered a following among individuals seeking alternative approaches to health and healing.

Eliminating Acidic Foods and Substances from the Diet

One of the fundamental principles of Dr. Sebi's alkaline diet approach to cancer is the elimination of acidic foods and substances from the diet. According to Dr. Sebi, acidic foods are believed to create an environment in the body that is conducive to disease development, including cancer. Acidic foods include animal products such as meat, dairy, and eggs, as well as processed foods, refined sugars, caffeine, alcohol, and artificial additives.

Dr. Sebi advocated for a plant-based diet consisting primarily of alkaline-rich foods, such as fruits, vegetables, nuts, seeds, grains, and legumes. These foods are believed to help maintain an alkaline pH balance in the body, which can support cellular health and immune function. By eliminating acidic foods and substances from the diet, individuals following Dr. Sebi's approach aim to create an internal environment that is less hospitable to cancer growth and proliferation.

Emphasizing Alkaline-Rich Foods for Cellular Health and Immune Support

Another key principle of Dr. Sebi's alkaline diet approach to cancer is the emphasis on alkaline-rich foods for cellular health and immune support. Alkaline-rich foods are those that have an alkalizing effect on the body when metabolized, helping to maintain a slightly alkaline pH balance in the blood and tissues. These foods are typically plant-based and are rich in vitamins, minerals, antioxidants, and phytonutrients that support overall health and well-being.

Some examples of alkaline-rich foods recommended by Dr. Sebi include leafy greens, cruciferous vegetables, root vegetables, fruits, nuts, seeds, grains, and legumes. These foods are believed to provide essential nutrients and antioxidants that can help protect cells from oxidative damage, support detoxification pathways, and enhance immune function. By incorporating alkaline-rich foods into their diet, individuals following Dr. Sebi's approach aim to nourish their bodies at the cellular level and strengthen their immune system's ability to defend against cancer and other diseases.

Understanding the Importance of Herbal Supplements in Cancer Management

In addition to dietary modifications, Dr. Sebi also emphasized the importance of herbal supplements in cancer management. Dr. Sebi believed that certain herbs and botanicals possess powerful healing properties that can support the body's natural ability to fight cancer and restore balance. These herbal supplements are often used in conjunction with dietary changes as part of a holistic approach to cancer prevention and treatment.

Some examples of herbal supplements recommended by Dr. Sebi for cancer management include burdock root, soursop, sea moss, bladderwrack, elderberry, and dandelion root. These herbs are believed to possess anti-inflammatory, antioxidant, immune-modulating, and anti-cancer properties that can help inhibit tumor growth, reduce inflammation, support detoxification, and enhance overall health and well-being.

While the use of herbal supplements in cancer management is a topic of ongoing research and debate, some studies have suggested potential benefits for certain herbs in cancer prevention and treatment. For example, research has shown that compounds found in herbs such as turmeric, green tea, and garlic may exhibit anti-cancer effects by inhibiting tumor cell proliferation, promoting apoptosis (cell death), and modulating inflammatory pathways. However, more rigorous clinical trials are needed to evaluate the safety and efficacy of herbal supplements in cancer management and to determine their optimal dosing and use in clinical practice.

In conclusion, Dr. Sebi's alkaline diet approach to cancer is based on the principles of eliminating acidic foods, emphasizing alkaline-rich foods for cellular health and immune support, and incorporating herbal supplements to support cancer management. While his methods and claims have been met with skepticism, some individuals may find value in adopting a plant-based, alkaline-rich diet and incorporating herbal supplements as part of a holistic approach to cancer prevention and treatment. As with any dietary or lifestyle intervention, it is essential to consult with healthcare professionals before making significant changes, especially for individuals with cancer or other underlying health conditions.

BOOK 2

Alkaline Foods and Their Anti-Cancer Properties

In the realm of nutrition and cancer prevention, alkaline foods have garnered attention for their potential anti-cancer properties. Alkaline foods, which include various vegetables, fruits, and herbs, are believed to help maintain the body's pH balance, support detoxification processes, and provide essential nutrients and phytochemicals that may help reduce cancer risk and inhibit tumor growth. Understanding the specific properties of alkaline foods and their potential effects on cancer can provide valuable insights into dietary strategies for cancer prevention and treatment.

Alkaline Vegetables for Detoxification and Nutrient Replenishment

Alkaline vegetables play a crucial role in maintaining the body's pH balance and supporting overall health. These vegetables are rich in essential vitamins, minerals, antioxidants, and dietary fiber, which contribute to various physiological processes, including detoxification and nutrient replenishment. Some examples of alkaline vegetables with potential anti-cancer properties include:

- Cruciferous Vegetables: Cruciferous vegetables such as broccoli, kale, cabbage, Brussels sprouts, and cauliflower are rich in glucosinolates, sulfur-containing compounds that have been shown to possess anti-cancer properties. Studies suggest that glucosinolates may help inhibit cancer cell growth, promote apoptosis (cell death), and modulate inflammatory pathways. Additionally, cruciferous vegetables are excellent sources of vitamin C, vitamin K, folate, and fiber, which support immune function and digestive health.

- Leafy Greens: Leafy green vegetables such as spinach, Swiss chard, collard greens, and arugula are alkaline-rich foods that are packed with nutrients and antioxidants. These vegetables are particularly rich in chlorophyll, a green pigment with detoxifying properties that may help eliminate toxins and carcinogens from the body. Additionally, leafy greens are high in vitamins A, C, and K, as well as minerals like magnesium and potassium, which support cellular health and immune function.

- Root Vegetables: Root vegetables such as carrots, sweet potatoes, beets, and radishes are alkaline-rich foods that provide a diverse array of nutrients and phytochemicals. These vegetables are rich in beta-carotene, a precursor to vitamin A, which exhibits antioxidant properties that may help protect cells from oxidative damage. Additionally, root vegetables are high in dietary fiber, which supports digestive health and may help reduce the risk of colorectal cancer.

Incorporating a variety of alkaline vegetables into the diet can help support detoxification processes, replenish essential nutrients, and reduce cancer risk by providing a diverse array of phytochemicals with potential anti-cancer properties.

Alkaline Fruits with Antioxidant and Anti-inflammatory Benefits

Alkaline fruits are another important component of a cancer-preventive diet due to their antioxidant and anti-inflammatory properties. These fruits are rich in vitamins, minerals, antioxidants, and phytochemicals that may help reduce oxidative stress, inflammation, and cancer risk. Some examples of alkaline fruits with potential anti-cancer benefits include:

- Berries: Berries such as strawberries, blueberries, raspberries, and blackberries are alkaline-rich foods that are packed with antioxidants, including vitamin C, flavonoids, and anthocyanins. These compounds have been shown to possess anti-inflammatory and anti-cancer properties, inhibiting tumor growth and reducing oxidative damage to cells. Additionally, berries are high in dietary fiber, which supports digestive health and may help reduce the risk of gastrointestinal cancers.

- Citrus Fruits: Citrus fruits such as oranges, lemons, limes, and grapefruits are alkaline-rich foods that are rich in vitamin C, a potent antioxidant that helps neutralize free radicals and protect cells from oxidative damage. Additionally, citrus fruits contain bioactive compounds such as limonoids and flavonoids, which have been shown to possess anti-cancer properties by inhibiting cancer cell proliferation and inducing apoptosis. Citrus fruits are also high in fiber, which supports digestive health and may help reduce the risk of colorectal cancer.

- Tropical Fruits: Tropical fruits such as papaya, pineapple, mango, and kiwi are alkaline-rich foods that provide a rich source of vitamins, minerals, and antioxidants. These fruits are particularly rich in vitamin C, vitamin A, and enzymes such as bromelain and papain, which have been shown to possess anti-inflammatory and anti-cancer properties. Additionally, tropical fruits are high in dietary fiber, which supports digestive health and may help reduce the risk of gastrointestinal cancers.

Incorporating a variety of alkaline fruits into the diet can help reduce oxidative stress, inflammation, and cancer risk by providing essential nutrients and phytochemicals with potential anti-cancer properties.

Alkaline Herbs for Targeted Cancer Therapy and Immune Support

Alkaline herbs have long been used in traditional medicine systems for their potential therapeutic properties, including cancer prevention and treatment. These herbs contain bioactive compounds such as polyphenols, flavonoids, terpenoids, and alkaloids, which have been shown to possess anti-inflammatory, antioxidant, and anti-cancer properties. Some examples of alkaline herbs with potential anti-cancer benefits include:

- Turmeric: Turmeric is an alkaline-rich herb that contains the bioactive compound curcumin, which has been extensively studied for its anti-inflammatory and anti-cancer properties. Curcumin has been shown to inhibit cancer cell proliferation, induce apoptosis, and modulate inflammatory pathways involved in cancer development and progression. Additionally, turmeric has been shown to enhance the efficacy of conventional cancer treatments, such as chemotherapy and radiation therapy, by sensitizing cancer cells to treatment-induced cell death.

- Ginger: Ginger is an alkaline-rich herb that contains bioactive compounds such as gingerol and shogaol, which have been shown to possess anti-inflammatory and anti-cancer properties. Ginger has been shown to inhibit cancer cell growth, induce apoptosis, and suppress tumor angiogenesis and metastasis in preclinical studies. Additionally, ginger has been shown to alleviate chemotherapy-induced nausea and vomiting and enhance the efficacy of chemotherapy in animal models of cancer.

- Garlic: Garlic is an alkaline-rich herb that contains bioactive compounds such as allicin, diallyl sulfide, and diallyl disulfide, which have been shown to possess anti-inflammatory, antioxidant, and anti-cancer properties. Garlic has been shown to inhibit cancer cell proliferation, induce apoptosis, and modulate inflammatory pathways involved in cancer development and progression. Additionally, garlic has been shown to enhance immune function and support detoxification processes, which may help reduce cancer risk and improve cancer outcomes.

Incorporating alkaline herbs into the diet can help support targeted cancer therapy, enhance immune function, and reduce inflammation and oxidative stress associated with cancer development and progression.

In conclusion, alkaline foods such as vegetables, fruits, and herbs offer a diverse array of nutrients and phytochemicals with potential anti-cancer properties. By incorporating alkaline-rich foods into the diet, individuals can help support detoxification processes, reduce oxidative stress and inflammation, and enhance immune function, thereby reducing cancer risk and improving overall health and well-being.

Dr. Sebi's Recommended Alkaline Diet Plan for Cancer Patients

Dr. Sebi's alkaline diet plan for cancer patients is based on the principles of eliminating acidic foods, emphasizing alkaline-rich foods, and incorporating herbal supplements to support healing and overall well-being. While Dr. Sebi's recommendations have been met with controversy and skepticism, some individuals may find value in adopting a plant-based, alkaline-rich diet as part of a holistic approach to cancer prevention and support.

Daily Meal Plans and Recipes for Cancer Prevention and Support

Dr. Sebi's alkaline diet plan for cancer patients emphasizes the consumption of alkaline-rich foods such as fruits, vegetables, nuts, seeds, grains, and legumes, while eliminating or minimizing acidic foods such as meat, dairy, processed foods, refined sugars, caffeine, alcohol, and artificial additives. Here's a sample daily meal plan based on Dr. Sebi's recommendations:

- Breakfast: Start the day with a nutrient-rich smoothie made with alkaline fruits such as berries, bananas, and mangoes, along with leafy greens like spinach or kale, and a tablespoon of chia seeds or flaxseeds for added fiber and omega-3 fatty acids.

- Mid-Morning Snack: Enjoy a handful of raw almonds or walnuts for a satisfying and nutritious snack that provides essential vitamins, minerals, and healthy fats.

- Lunch: For lunch, prepare a colorful salad with mixed greens, bell peppers, cucumbers, tomatoes, avocado, and chickpeas or lentils for protein. Dress the salad with a simple vinaigrette made with olive oil, lemon juice, and herbs.

- Afternoon Snack: Have a piece of fresh fruit such as an apple, pear, or orange, or enjoy sliced vegetables with hummus for a satisfying and energizing snack.

- Dinner: For dinner, prepare a hearty vegetable stir-fry with alkaline vegetables such as broccoli, bell peppers, carrots, and mushrooms, served over quinoa or brown rice for a complete and balanced meal.

Guidelines for Meal Timing and Portion Control to Support Healing

In addition to emphasizing alkaline-rich foods, Dr. Sebi's alkaline diet plan for cancer patients also includes guidelines for meal timing and portion control to support healing and optimal health. Here are some general recommendations:

- Eat Regularly: Aim to eat regular meals and snacks throughout the day to maintain stable blood sugar levels and provide your body with a steady supply of nutrients and energy.

- Practice Mindful Eating: Pay attention to hunger and fullness cues, and eat slowly and mindfully to allow your body to digest food properly and optimize nutrient absorption.

- Portion Control: Be mindful of portion sizes and avoid overeating, especially high-calorie or high-fat foods, to prevent weight gain and promote overall health.

- Stay Hydrated: Drink plenty of water throughout the day to stay hydrated and support detoxification processes. Herbal teas and fresh juices can also be included as part of your hydration plan.

Incorporating Juicing and Smoothies into the Alkaline Diet for Enhanced Nutrient Absorption

Juicing and smoothies can be valuable additions to Dr. Sebi's alkaline diet plan for cancer patients, as they provide a convenient and delicious way to increase your intake of alkaline-rich foods and enhance nutrient absorption. Here are some tips for incorporating juicing and smoothies into your daily routine:

- Include a Variety of Ingredients: Experiment with different combinations of fruits, vegetables, leafy greens, herbs, and superfoods to create nutrient-dense and flavorful juices and smoothies.

- Focus on Fresh, Organic Produce: Whenever possible, choose fresh, organic produce to maximize nutrient content and minimize exposure to pesticides and other harmful chemicals.

- Add Healthy Fats and Proteins: To make your juices and smoothies more satisfying and balanced, consider adding sources of healthy fats and proteins such as avocado, nuts, seeds, nut butter, or plant-based protein powder.

- Drink Immediately or Store Properly: Freshly prepared juices and smoothies are best consumed immediately to preserve nutrient integrity and flavor. If you need to store them for later, use airtight containers and refrigerate promptly to minimize nutrient loss and bacterial growth.

In conclusion, Dr. Sebi's alkaline diet plan for cancer patients emphasizes the consumption of alkaline-rich foods, herbal supplements, and hydration to support healing and overall well-being. By following guidelines for meal planning, timing, portion control, and incorporating juicing and smoothies, individuals can optimize nutrient absorption and promote optimal health and vitality during cancer prevention and support. As always, it is essential to consult with healthcare professionals before making significant dietary changes, especially for individuals with cancer or other underlying health conditions.

Alkaline Diet and Lifestyle Changes for Specific Types of Cancer

When it comes to cancer prevention and support, dietary and lifestyle factors play a significant role in influencing overall health and well-being. The alkaline diet, with its emphasis on consuming alkaline-forming foods and minimizing acidic foods, may offer potential benefits for individuals at risk of or diagnosed with certain types of cancer. In this section, we'll explore specific strategies for breast cancer prevention and support, prostate cancer management and prevention, and colon cancer prevention and treatment within the context of the alkaline diet.

Alkaline Diet Strategies for Breast Cancer Prevention and Support

Breast cancer is one of the most common cancers affecting women worldwide, and lifestyle factors, including diet, play a crucial role in its prevention and management. While there is no single "magic bullet" for preventing breast cancer, adopting a plant-based, alkaline-rich diet may offer protective benefits. Here are some alkaline diet strategies for breast cancer prevention and support:

- Emphasize Plant-Based Foods: Focus on consuming a variety of fruits, vegetables, nuts, seeds, legumes, and whole grains, which are alkaline-forming and rich in vitamins, minerals, antioxidants, and phytochemicals that may help reduce breast cancer risk.

- Limit Animal Products: Minimize the consumption of red and processed meats, dairy products, and other acidic foods, as these may increase inflammation and oxidative stress, contributing to breast cancer development and progression.

- Choose Healthy Fats: Opt for sources of healthy fats such as avocados, nuts, seeds, and olive oil, which provide essential fatty acids and antioxidants that may help reduce breast cancer risk.

- Stay Hydrated: Drink plenty of water throughout the day to stay hydrated and support detoxification processes. Herbal teas and fresh juices can also be included as part of your hydration plan.

In addition to dietary changes, other lifestyle factors such as regular physical activity, maintaining a healthy weight, limiting alcohol consumption, and avoiding exposure to environmental toxins can also help reduce breast cancer risk and support overall health and well-being.

Alkaline Foods for Prostate Cancer Management and Prevention

Prostate cancer is the most common cancer affecting men worldwide, and dietary factors may play a role in its development and progression. While more research is needed to fully understand the relationship between diet and prostate cancer, adopting an alkaline-rich diet may offer potential benefits. Here are some alkaline diet approaches for prostate cancer management and prevention:

- Eat Plenty of Fruits and Vegetables: Incorporate a variety of fruits and vegetables into your diet, including leafy greens, cruciferous vegetables, tomatoes, berries, and citrus fruits, which are rich in antioxidants, vitamins, minerals, and phytochemicals that may help reduce prostate cancer risk.

- Choose Plant-Based Proteins: Opt for plant-based sources of protein such as legumes, tofu, tempeh, and quinoa, which are alkaline-forming and may help reduce inflammation and oxidative stress associated with prostate cancer.

- Include Healthy Fats: Include sources of healthy fats such as avocados, nuts, seeds, and olive oil, which provide essential fatty acids and antioxidants that may help reduce prostate cancer risk.

- Limit Red and Processed Meats: Minimize the consumption of red and processed meats, which are acidic and may increase inflammation and oxidative stress, contributing to prostate cancer development and progression.

In addition to dietary changes, maintaining a healthy weight, staying physically active, managing stress, and avoiding tobacco products can also help reduce prostate cancer risk and support overall health and well-being.

Alkaline Diet Approaches for Colon Cancer Prevention and Treatment

Colon cancer is one of the most common cancers worldwide, and diet plays a crucial role in its prevention and treatment. Adopting an alkaline-rich diet may offer potential benefits for colon cancer prevention and support. Here are some alkaline diet approaches for colon cancer prevention and treatment:

- Eat Plenty of Fiber-Rich Foods: Include a variety of fiber-rich foods in your diet, such as fruits, vegetables, whole grains, legumes, and nuts, which are alkaline-forming and may help promote regular bowel movements and reduce colon cancer risk.

- Choose Whole Grains: Opt for whole grains such as brown rice, quinoa, oats, and barley, which are rich in fiber, vitamins, minerals, and antioxidants that may help reduce colon cancer risk.

- Limit Red and Processed Meats: Minimize the consumption of red and processed meats, which are acidic and may increase inflammation and oxidative stress, contributing to colon cancer development and progression.

- Stay Hydrated: Drink plenty of water throughout the day to stay hydrated and support digestive health. Herbal teas and fresh juices can also be included as part of your hydration plan.

In addition to dietary changes, regular physical activity, maintaining a healthy weight, avoiding tobacco products, and participating in regular screening tests can also help reduce colon cancer risk and support overall health and well-being.

In conclusion, adopting an alkaline-rich diet and making lifestyle changes such as maintaining a healthy weight, staying physically active, managing stress, and avoiding tobacco products can help reduce the risk of certain types of cancer and support overall health and well-being. As always, it is essential to consult with healthcare professionals before making significant dietary changes, especially for individuals with cancer or other underlying health conditions.

BOOK 3

Addressing Challenges and Side Effects on the Alkaline Diet for Cancer

Following an alkaline diet for cancer can be beneficial for some individuals, but it may also present challenges and side effects. In this section, we'll explore strategies for coping with detox symptoms and cleansing reactions, managing nutritional needs and dietary restrictions during cancer treatment, and overcoming social and practical challenges of the alkaline diet.

Coping with Detox Symptoms and Cleansing Reactions

When transitioning to an alkaline diet, some individuals may experience detox symptoms and cleansing reactions as their bodies adjust to dietary changes and eliminate toxins. These symptoms may include headaches, fatigue, digestive disturbances, skin breakouts, and mood changes. Here are some strategies for coping with detox symptoms and cleansing reactions:

- Stay Hydrated: Drink plenty of water throughout the day to support detoxification processes and help flush out toxins from the body.

- Gradual Transition: Gradually transition to an alkaline diet by slowly reducing acidic foods and increasing alkaline-rich foods over time to minimize detox symptoms.

- Supportive Therapies: Consider incorporating supportive therapies such as massage, acupuncture, dry brushing, and sauna therapy to help facilitate detoxification and alleviate detox symptoms.

- Listen to Your Body: Pay attention to your body's signals and adjust your diet and lifestyle as needed to support your individual needs and preferences.

- Consult with a Healthcare Professional: If detox symptoms persist or become severe, consult with a healthcare professional for personalized guidance and support.

Managing Nutritional Needs and Dietary Restrictions During Cancer Treatment

During cancer treatment, such as chemotherapy, radiation therapy, or surgery, individuals may experience changes in appetite, taste preferences, digestion, and nutrient absorption, making it challenging to meet their nutritional needs. Here are some strategies for managing nutritional needs and dietary restrictions during cancer treatment:

- Work with a Registered Dietitian: Consult with a registered dietitian who specializes in oncology nutrition to develop a personalized nutrition plan that meets your specific needs and dietary restrictions during cancer treatment.

- Focus on Nutrient-Dense Foods: Prioritize nutrient-dense foods such as fruits, vegetables, whole grains, lean proteins, and healthy fats to ensure adequate intake of essential nutrients during cancer treatment.

- Optimize Digestion: Choose easily digestible foods and cooking methods, such as steaming, boiling, baking, and blending, to minimize digestive discomfort and promote nutrient absorption.

- Consider Nutritional Supplements: In some cases, nutritional supplements such as protein powders, meal replacement shakes, vitamin and mineral supplements, and herbal supplements may be recommended to address nutrient deficiencies and support overall health during cancer treatment.

- Communicate with Your Healthcare Team: Keep open communication with your healthcare team, including oncologists, nurses, and dietitians, to address any concerns or challenges related to nutrition and dietary restrictions during cancer treatment.

Strategies for Overcoming Social and Practical Challenges of the Alkaline Diet

Following an alkaline diet may present social and practical challenges, such as dining out, attending social gatherings, traveling, and grocery shopping. Here are some strategies for overcoming social and practical challenges of the alkaline diet:

- Plan Ahead: Plan your meals and snacks in advance, and consider bringing your own alkaline-friendly dishes to social gatherings or events.

- Communicate with Others: Communicate your dietary preferences and restrictions with friends, family members, and restaurant staff to ensure accommodations can be made when dining out or attending social gatherings.

- Be Flexible: Be flexible and creative with your food choices, and focus on enjoying the company of others rather than solely on dietary restrictions.

- Seek Support: Join online forums, support groups, or social media communities for individuals following an alkaline diet to connect with others, share experiences, and exchange tips and recipes.

- Focus on Health and Well-being: Remember that the primary goal of following an alkaline diet is to support your health and well-being, so prioritize self-care and stress management practices to maintain balance and perspective.

In conclusion, while following an alkaline diet for cancer may offer potential benefits, it is essential to be mindful of potential challenges and side effects and to adopt strategies for coping with detox symptoms and cleansing reactions, managing nutritional needs and dietary restrictions during cancer treatment, and overcoming social and practical challenges. As always, consult with a healthcare professional before making significant dietary changes, especially for individuals with cancer or other underlying health conditions.

Success Stories and Testimonials of Cancer Healing with Dr. Sebi's Alkaline Diet

Real-Life Accounts of Cancer Remission Through the Alkaline Diet

Numerous individuals have shared their experiences of cancer remission and improved health outcomes through the adoption of Dr. Sebi's alkaline diet. While anecdotal evidence cannot substitute for scientific research, these personal accounts provide insights into the potential impact of dietary changes on cancer healing. Here are a few real-life stories of cancer remission through the alkaline diet:

1. Mary's Story: Mary was diagnosed with breast cancer and underwent conventional treatments, including surgery, chemotherapy, and radiation therapy. Despite these interventions, her cancer continued to progress. Desperate for alternative options, Mary decided to explore dietary changes and began following Dr. Sebi's alkaline diet. Over time, Mary noticed significant improvements in her energy levels, digestion, and overall well-being. Her follow-up scans revealed a reduction in tumor size and ultimately, her cancer went into remission.

2. John's Story: John was diagnosed with prostate cancer and was facing surgery as the primary treatment option. Concerned about the potential side effects and complications of surgery, John decided to explore holistic approaches to cancer treatment. He began following Dr. Sebi's alkaline diet, focusing on alkaline-rich foods and herbal supplements. Within a few months, John's PSA levels, a marker for prostate cancer, began to decline, and his follow-up biopsies showed a reduction in tumor size. Today, John remains cancer-free and attributes his success to the alkaline diet and lifestyle changes.

3. Sarah's Story: Sarah was diagnosed with colon cancer and underwent surgery to remove the tumor. However, her cancer returned, and she was advised to undergo

chemotherapy and radiation therapy. Concerned about the potential side effects and toxicity of conventional treatments, Sarah decided to explore alternative approaches to cancer healing. She began following Dr. Sebi's alkaline diet and incorporated juicing and herbal supplements into her daily routine. Over time, Sarah experienced improvements in her symptoms, and her follow-up scans showed no evidence of cancer recurrence.

How the Alkaline Diet Transformed Lives and Improved Cancer Outcomes

The alkaline diet has transformed the lives of many individuals diagnosed with cancer, offering hope and healing where conventional treatments alone may have fallen short. While the scientific evidence supporting the alkaline diet's efficacy in cancer treatment is still evolving, these personal testimonials highlight the potential benefits of dietary changes in improving cancer outcomes. Here are some ways in which the alkaline diet has transformed lives and improved cancer outcomes:

1. Enhanced Quality of Life: Many individuals following the alkaline diet report improvements in their quality of life, including increased energy levels, better digestion, improved mood, and reduced pain and inflammation. These improvements can have a profound impact on overall well-being and resilience during cancer treatment and recovery.

2. Reduced Side Effects of Treatment: The alkaline diet may help reduce the side effects and toxicity associated with conventional cancer treatments such as chemotherapy and radiation therapy. By supporting detoxification processes, reducing inflammation, and enhancing immune function, the alkaline diet can help mitigate treatment-related side effects and improve tolerance to therapy.

3. Supportive Care and Symptom Management: In addition to its potential role in cancer treatment, the alkaline diet can also serve as a valuable adjunctive therapy for supportive care and symptom management. By focusing on nutrient-dense, anti-inflammatory foods and herbal supplements, individuals can support their bodies' natural healing processes and alleviate symptoms associated with cancer and its treatment.

Inspiring Stories of Cancer Survival and Thriving on the Alkaline Diet

Despite the challenges of a cancer diagnosis, many individuals have found inspiration and hope through their journey with the alkaline diet. These stories of cancer survival and thriving on the alkaline diet serve as a testament to the power of dietary changes in promoting healing and resilience. Here are some inspiring stories of cancer survival and thriving on the alkaline diet:

1. James' Journey: James was diagnosed with pancreatic cancer, one of the deadliest forms of cancer with limited treatment options and poor prognosis. Determined to defy the odds, James embraced the alkaline diet and made radical changes to his lifestyle. Through a combination of dietary changes, juicing, herbal supplements, and mind-body practices, James not only survived his cancer diagnosis but thrived, becoming an advocate for holistic approaches to cancer healing.

2. Lisa's Triumph: Lisa was diagnosed with ovarian cancer and underwent surgery followed by chemotherapy. Despite aggressive treatment, her cancer persisted, and she was given a grim prognosis. Refusing to accept defeat, Lisa embarked on a journey of healing with the alkaline diet and lifestyle changes. Over time, her cancer markers normalized, and her follow-up scans showed no evidence of disease. Today, Lisa continues to enjoy a vibrant and healthy life, inspiring others with her story of triumph over cancer.

3. David's Resilience: David was diagnosed with lung cancer and was told he had only months to live. Determined to fight for his life, David embraced the alkaline diet and herbal remedies, alongside conventional treatments. Despite the odds, David's cancer responded positively to his holistic approach, and he experienced significant improvements in

his health and well-being. Today, David remains cancer-free and cherishes each day as a gift of life.

In conclusion, the alkaline diet has offered hope and healing to many individuals diagnosed with cancer, with numerous success stories and testimonials highlighting its potential benefits in promoting cancer remission, improving quality of life, and inspiring resilience. While more research is needed to fully understand the role of the alkaline diet in cancer treatment and prevention, these personal accounts serve as powerful reminders of the transformative power of dietary changes in cancer healing.

BOOK 4

Integrating Dr. Sebi's Alkaline Diet with Conventional Cancer Treatment

Collaboration with Oncologists and Healthcare Providers for Comprehensive Care

Integrating Dr. Sebi's alkaline diet with conventional cancer treatment involves collaboration between patients, oncologists, and healthcare providers to ensure comprehensive care. Open communication and mutual respect between all parties are essential for developing a cohesive treatment plan that addresses the individual's unique needs and preferences. Here are some key considerations for collaboration:

1. Open Dialogue: Patients should openly communicate their interest in incorporating the alkaline diet into their cancer treatment plan with their oncologist and healthcare team. Oncologists, in turn, should be receptive to their patients' preferences and concerns and be willing to discuss the potential benefits and risks of dietary changes.

2. Shared Decision-Making: Treatment decisions should be made collaboratively, taking into account the patient's preferences, medical history, cancer stage, treatment goals, and potential interactions between the alkaline diet and conventional therapies. Healthcare providers should provide

evidence-based information and support patients in making informed decisions about their care.

3. Monitoring and Follow-Up: Patients following an alkaline diet should be monitored closely by their healthcare team to assess their response to treatment, nutritional status, and overall well-being. Regular follow-up appointments allow healthcare providers to address any concerns or complications that may arise and make adjustments to the treatment plan as needed.

Combining Alkaline Diet Principles with Chemotherapy and Radiation Therapy

Integrating Dr. Sebi's alkaline diet principles with chemotherapy and radiation therapy requires careful consideration of potential interactions and synergies between dietary changes and medical treatments. While more research is needed to fully understand the impact of the alkaline diet on cancer treatment outcomes, some individuals may choose to incorporate alkaline-rich foods into their diet alongside conventional therapies. Here are some considerations for combining the alkaline diet with chemotherapy and radiation therapy:

1. Nutritional Support: Chemotherapy and radiation therapy can place additional stress on the body and compromise nutritional status. The alkaline diet, with its emphasis on nutrient-dense, anti-inflammatory foods, may help support

immune function, reduce inflammation, and mitigate treatment-related side effects such as nausea, fatigue, and digestive disturbances.

2. Timing of Meals: Patients undergoing chemotherapy and radiation therapy should pay attention to the timing of meals and avoid consuming acidic or potentially irritating foods immediately before or after treatment sessions. Opting for alkaline-rich foods such as fruits, vegetables, whole grains, and plant-based proteins can help maintain stable blood sugar levels and provide sustained energy throughout the treatment process.

3. Hydration: Staying hydrated is essential during cancer treatment to support detoxification processes, maintain electrolyte balance, and prevent dehydration. Patients following an alkaline diet should prioritize water intake and avoid sugary or caffeinated beverages, which can contribute to acidity and dehydration.

Using Herbal Supplements as Complementary Therapy in Conjunction with Medical Treatment

Herbal supplements can serve as complementary therapy alongside conventional cancer treatment, providing additional support for immune function, detoxification, and overall well-being. While some herbal supplements may interact with chemotherapy or radiation therapy, others may complement medical treatments and enhance their effectiveness. Here are some considerations for using herbal supplements in conjunction with medical treatment:

1. Consultation with Healthcare Providers: Patients should consult with their oncologist or healthcare provider before starting any herbal supplements to ensure safety and avoid potential interactions with chemotherapy or radiation therapy. Healthcare providers can provide guidance on suitable supplements, appropriate dosages, and potential side effects.

2. Quality and Safety: Patients should choose high-quality herbal supplements from reputable sources to ensure purity, potency, and safety. Look for supplements that have been independently tested for quality and consistency and adhere to good manufacturing practices (GMP).

3. Individualized Approach: Herbal supplements should be selected based on the individual's specific cancer type, treatment regimen, medical history, and overall health status. Some herbal supplements with potential anticancer properties include turmeric, ginger, green tea, garlic, and medicinal mushrooms such as reishi and maitake.

In conclusion, integrating Dr. Sebi's alkaline diet with conventional cancer treatment requires collaboration between patients, oncologists, and healthcare providers to ensure comprehensive care and optimize treatment outcomes. By fostering open communication, shared decision-making, and a personalized approach to care, patients can harness the potential benefits of the alkaline diet while receiving evidence-based medical treatments for cancer. As always, it is essential to consult with healthcare professionals before making significant dietary changes or starting any herbal supplements, especially for individuals undergoing cancer treatment.

Frequently Asked Questions about Dr. Sebi's Alkaline Diet for Cancer

Addressing Common Concerns and Misconceptions about the Alkaline Diet

Q: Is the alkaline diet a cure for cancer? A: The alkaline diet is not a cure for cancer on its own. While some proponents believe that maintaining an alkaline environment in the body can prevent or treat cancer, scientific evidence supporting this claim is limited. However, the alkaline diet can be part of a holistic approach to cancer prevention and support, alongside conventional medical treatments.

Q: Are there any risks associated with the alkaline diet? A: Like any dietary approach, the alkaline diet may pose risks for certain individuals, particularly those with underlying health conditions or specific dietary needs. Risks may include nutrient deficiencies, inadequate calorie intake, and potential interactions with medications or medical treatments. It's essential to consult with a healthcare professional before making significant dietary changes, especially for individuals with cancer.

Q: Can the alkaline diet alkalize the body? A: The body's pH balance is tightly regulated by physiological mechanisms, and dietary changes alone are unlikely to significantly alter blood pH. However, the alkaline diet emphasizes consuming alkaline-forming foods that may have alkalizing effects on urine pH. While urine pH can be influenced by diet, it does not necessarily reflect the body's overall pH balance or health status.

Practical Tips for Adhering to the Alkaline Diet While Managing Cancer

Q: How can I incorporate more alkaline-rich foods into my diet? A: To incorporate more alkaline-rich foods into your diet, focus on consuming a variety of fruits, vegetables, nuts, seeds, legumes, and whole grains. Aim to fill half of your plate with alkaline foods at each meal and experiment with different recipes and cooking methods to make them more enjoyable.

Q: Are there any convenient alkaline snacks I can keep on hand? A: Yes, there are many convenient alkaline snacks you can keep on hand, such as raw nuts and seeds, fresh fruit, chopped vegetables with hummus, whole grain crackers with avocado, or homemade trail mix with dried fruits and nuts. These snacks are portable, nutritious, and easy to incorporate into your daily routine.

Q: How can I stay motivated to stick to the alkaline diet during cancer treatment? A: Staying motivated to stick to the alkaline diet during cancer treatment can be challenging, but it's essential to focus on the potential benefits for your health and well-being. Surround yourself with supportive friends and family members, set realistic goals, celebrate small victories, and seek inspiration from success stories and testimonials of others who have thrived on the alkaline diet.

Seeking Professional Guidance and Support for Implementing the Alkaline Diet in Cancer Care

Q: Should I consult with a healthcare professional before starting the alkaline diet for cancer? A: Yes, it's essential to consult with a healthcare professional before starting the alkaline diet for cancer, especially if you're undergoing medical treatment or have underlying health conditions. A registered dietitian, oncologist, or integrative healthcare provider can provide personalized guidance and support based on your individual needs and medical history.

Q: Are there any specialized oncology dietitians who can help me with the alkaline diet? A: Yes, many oncology dietitians specialize in providing nutrition counseling and support for individuals with cancer. These professionals can help you develop a personalized nutrition plan that aligns with your treatment goals, dietary preferences, and lifestyle factors while considering the principles of the alkaline diet.

Q: Can I find support groups or online communities for individuals following the alkaline diet for cancer? A: Yes, there are many support groups and online communities for individuals following the alkaline diet for cancer where you can connect with others, share experiences, exchange tips and recipes, and find inspiration and encouragement. These communities can provide valuable support and camaraderie on your journey to better health.

Continuing the Journey to Cancer Wellness with Dr. Sebi's Alkaline Diet

Long-Term Strategies for Maintaining Health and Preventing Cancer Recurrence

Maintaining health and preventing cancer recurrence require long-term commitment and ongoing lifestyle adjustments. Dr. Sebi's alkaline diet can be an integral part of a holistic approach to cancer wellness. Here are some long-term strategies for maintaining health and preventing cancer recurrence with the alkaline diet:

1. **Consistency is Key:** Stay consistent with your alkaline diet by incorporating alkaline-rich foods into your daily meals and snacks. Consistency over time can help maintain optimal pH balance in the body and support overall health.

2. **Regular Monitoring:** Continue to monitor your health closely with regular check-ups, screenings, and follow-up appointments with your healthcare team. Early detection of any potential issues can lead to prompt intervention and better outcomes.

3. **Stay Active:** Regular physical activity is essential for maintaining a healthy weight, supporting immune function, and reducing the risk of cancer recurrence. Aim for at least 150 minutes of moderate-intensity exercise per week, such as brisk walking, swimming, or cycling.

4. **Stress Management:** Chronic stress can weaken the immune system and contribute to inflammation, which may increase the risk of cancer recurrence. Practice stress management techniques such as mindfulness meditation, deep breathing exercises, yoga, or tai chi to promote relaxation and well-being.

5. **Limit Environmental Exposures:** Minimize exposure to environmental toxins and pollutants that may contribute to cancer risk. Choose organic produce whenever possible,

avoid tobacco smoke, limit alcohol consumption, and use natural, non-toxic household and personal care products.

6. **Quality Sleep:** Prioritize quality sleep by maintaining a regular sleep schedule, creating a relaxing bedtime routine, and optimizing your sleep environment. Aim for 7-9 hours of uninterrupted sleep per night to support immune function and overall health.

7. **Stay Informed:** Stay informed about the latest research and recommendations for cancer prevention and wellness. Attend educational workshops, seminars, or webinars, and seek out reputable sources of information to empower yourself with knowledge about cancer prevention and healthy living.

Building a Supportive Community and Network for Alkaline Diet Adherents

Building a supportive community and network of like-minded individuals can provide encouragement, accountability, and camaraderie on your journey to cancer wellness with the alkaline diet. Here are some ways to build a supportive community:

1. **Join Support Groups:** Seek out local or online support groups for individuals following the alkaline diet for cancer wellness. These groups can provide a platform for sharing experiences,

exchanging tips and recipes, and offering emotional support to one another.

2. **Connect with Others:** Reach out to friends, family members, or colleagues who may share an interest in holistic approaches to health and wellness, including the alkaline diet. Share your journey with them, invite them to join you in preparing alkaline meals, and celebrate your successes together.

3. **Attend Workshops or Events:** Attend workshops, seminars, or events focused on holistic health, nutrition, and cancer wellness. These gatherings can provide opportunities to connect with like-minded individuals, learn from experts in the field, and expand your knowledge and skills.

4. **Utilize Online Resources:** Take advantage of online resources such as forums, social media groups, and blogs dedicated to the alkaline diet and cancer wellness. Engage with others in these virtual communities, ask questions, and share your experiences and insights.

5. **Volunteer or Advocate:** Consider volunteering with organizations or advocacy groups that promote cancer awareness, prevention, and support. By giving back to your community and raising awareness about the benefits of the alkaline diet for cancer wellness, you can make a positive impact and inspire others to prioritize their health.

Embracing a Holistic Lifestyle Beyond Diet for Overall Wellbeing and Cancer Prevention

While the alkaline diet is an essential component of cancer wellness, embracing a holistic lifestyle goes beyond diet and encompasses various aspects of physical, mental, and emotional well-being. Here are some holistic lifestyle practices to consider:

1. **Mind-Body Practices:** Incorporate mind-body practices such as meditation, yoga, tai chi, or qigong into your daily routine to promote relaxation, reduce stress, and enhance overall well-being. These practices can also support immune function and resilience during cancer treatment and recovery.

2. **Nature Connection:** Spend time in nature regularly by going for walks, hikes, or picnics in parks, forests, or gardens. Connecting with nature has been shown to reduce stress, improve mood, and enhance feelings of vitality and well-being.

3. **Creative Expression:** Engage in creative activities such as painting, writing, gardening, or playing music as a form of self-expression and stress relief. Creative expression can help foster a sense of purpose, meaning, and joy in life, which are essential for overall well-being.

4. **Social Connection:** Cultivate meaningful relationships with friends, family members, and community members who support and uplift you. Maintain regular social connections through phone calls, video chats, or in-person gatherings to combat feelings of isolation and loneliness.

5. **Spiritual Practices:** Explore spiritual practices such as prayer, meditation, or mindfulness to nurture your inner life and connect with a sense of purpose, meaning, and transcendence. Spiritual practices can provide comfort, guidance, and strength during challenging times and contribute to overall well-being.

In conclusion, continuing the journey to cancer wellness with Dr. Sebi's alkaline diet involves adopting long-term strategies for maintaining health, building a supportive community, and embracing a holistic lifestyle beyond diet. By incorporating these practices into your daily life, you can enhance your overall well-being, reduce the risk of cancer recurrence, and thrive on your journey to optimal health and wellness.

BOOK 5

CANCER DIETS

Nordic Diet:

Ingredients:

1. Fatty fish (e.g., salmon, mackerel, herring)

2. Whole grains (e.g., rye, barley, oats, quinoa)

3. Berries (e.g., lingonberries, blueberries, raspberries)

4. Root vegetables (e.g., carrots, potatoes, beets, turnips)

5. Cruciferous vegetables (e.g., broccoli, Brussels sprouts, cabbage)

6. Leafy greens (e.g., kale, spinach, Swiss chard)

7. Legumes (e.g., beans, lentils, chickpeas)

8. Low-fat dairy products (e.g., skyr, yogurt, cheese)

9. Nuts and seeds (e.g., almonds, walnuts, flaxseeds, chia seeds)

10.   Rapeseed oil (canola oil)

Instructions:

1. Prioritize fatty fish: Incorporate fatty fish such as salmon, mackerel, and herring into your diet regularly for their

omega-3 fatty acids, which support heart health and reduce inflammation.

2. Include whole grains: Choose whole grains like rye, barley, oats, and quinoa as sources of fiber and nutrients, which help regulate blood sugar levels and promote satiety.

3. Eat plenty of berries: Enjoy a variety of berries such as lingonberries, blueberries, and raspberries, which are rich in antioxidants and vitamins.

4. Incorporate root vegetables: Include root vegetables like carrots, potatoes, and beets, which provide essential nutrients and add sweetness and texture to meals.

5. Include cruciferous vegetables: Incorporate cruciferous vegetables such as broccoli, Brussels sprouts, and cabbage, which are rich in fiber, vitamins, and phytochemicals.

6. Eat leafy greens: Include leafy greens like kale, spinach, and Swiss chard as sources of vitamins, minerals, and antioxidants.

7. Include legumes: Incorporate legumes such as beans, lentils, and chickpeas as plant-based protein sources and sources of fiber, which promote fullness and digestive health.

8. Choose low-fat dairy: Opt for low-fat dairy products like skyr, yogurt, and cheese as sources of calcium and protein, while keeping saturated fat intake in check.

9. Enjoy nuts and seeds: Include nuts and seeds such as almonds, walnuts, flaxseeds, and chia seeds as sources of healthy fats, protein, and fiber.

10. Cook with rapeseed oil: Use rapeseed oil (canola oil) for cooking and salad dressings, as it is a source of unsaturated fats and has a favorable omega-3 to omega-6 fatty acid ratio.

Ornish Diet:

Ingredients:

1. Whole grains (e.g., brown rice, quinoa, oats, whole wheat)

2. Fruits (e.g., apples, oranges, berries, bananas)

3. Vegetables (e.g., leafy greens, broccoli, carrots, bell peppers)

4. Legumes (e.g., beans, lentils, chickpeas)

5. Soy products (e.g., tofu, tempeh, edamame)

6. Non-fat dairy products (e.g., skim milk, yogurt)

7. Fish (especially fatty fish like salmon, trout)

8. Skinless poultry (e.g., chicken, turkey)

9. Nuts and seeds (e.g., almonds, walnuts, flaxseeds, chia seeds)

10. Herbs and spices (e.g., garlic, ginger, turmeric, basil)

Instructions:

1. Focus on whole, plant-based foods: Base your meals around whole grains, fruits, vegetables, legumes, and soy products, which are rich in fiber, vitamins, minerals, and phytochemicals.

2. Minimize processed and refined foods: Limit consumption of processed and refined foods, including white flour, sugar, and artificial additives, which can contribute to chronic diseases and weight gain.

3. Choose low-fat dairy: Opt for non-fat dairy products like skim milk and yogurt to reduce saturated fat intake while still obtaining essential nutrients like calcium and protein.

4. Include fish and poultry: Incorporate fish, especially fatty fish like salmon and trout, and skinless poultry into your diet as sources of lean protein and omega-3 fatty acids.

5. Limit added fats: Minimize consumption of added fats and oils, choosing lean cooking methods like steaming, baking, and grilling instead of frying.

6. Use nuts and seeds sparingly: Enjoy nuts and seeds like almonds, walnuts, flaxseeds, and chia seeds in moderation as sources of healthy fats, protein, and fiber.

7. Flavor with herbs and spices: Use herbs and spices liberally to add flavor to meals without relying on excessive salt or unhealthy condiments.

8. Eat mindfully: Practice mindful eating by paying attention to hunger and fullness cues, savoring each bite, and eating slowly to prevent overeating.

9. Stay hydrated: Drink plenty of water throughout the day to stay hydrated and support overall health, especially when consuming a high-fiber diet.

10. Be physically active: Incorporate regular physical activity into your routine to support heart health, weight management, and overall well-being, in combination with a healthy diet.

By following these guidelines, you can successfully adhere to the Nordic or Ornish diets, promoting better health and well-being through balanced nutrition and healthy lifestyle choices. Remember to consult with a healthcare professional or registered dietitian for personalized guidance and support, especially if you have specific dietary needs or medical conditions.

Raw Food Diet:

Ingredients:

1. Fresh fruits (e.g., apples, bananas, berries, oranges)

2. Vegetables (e.g., leafy greens, carrots, cucumbers, bell peppers)

3. Nuts and seeds (e.g., almonds, cashews, sunflower seeds, chia seeds)

4. Sprouts (e.g., alfalfa sprouts, broccoli sprouts, bean sprouts)

5. Whole grains (e.g., quinoa, buckwheat, oats)

6. Raw dairy alternatives (e.g., almond milk, cashew cheese)

7. Raw honey or maple syrup (in moderation)

8. Cold-pressed oils (e.g., olive oil, coconut oil, flaxseed oil)

9. Sea vegetables (e.g., nori, dulse, kelp)

10. Raw superfoods (e.g., spirulina, chlorella, maca powder)

Instructions:

1. Emphasize raw fruits and vegetables: Base the majority of your meals on fresh fruits and vegetables, which are rich in vitamins, minerals, enzymes, and phytonutrients in their raw state.

2. Include nuts and seeds: Incorporate a variety of nuts and seeds into your diet for healthy fats, protein, and essential nutrients. Sprouting nuts and seeds can enhance their nutritional value.

3. Add sprouts: Include a variety of sprouts in your meals, such as alfalfa sprouts, broccoli sprouts, and bean sprouts, for added texture and nutrition.

4. Experiment with whole grains: Incorporate raw whole grains like quinoa, buckwheat, and oats into your diet as sources of fiber, protein, and complex carbohydrates.

5. Opt for raw dairy alternatives: Choose raw dairy alternatives like almond milk and cashew cheese instead of traditional dairy products for those following a raw food diet.

6. Use cold-pressed oils: Use cold-pressed oils like olive oil, coconut oil, and flaxseed oil in moderation to add flavor and healthy fats to salads and raw dishes.

7. Include sea vegetables: Add sea vegetables like nori, dulse, and kelp to your diet for their rich mineral content and unique flavors.

8. Sweeten with raw honey or maple syrup: Use raw honey or maple syrup sparingly as natural sweeteners in recipes or as toppings for fruit-based desserts.

9. Incorporate raw superfoods: Include raw superfoods like spirulina, chlorella, and maca powder in your diet for their concentrated nutrients and potential health benefits.

10. Stay hydrated: Drink plenty of water throughout the day to stay hydrated, especially when consuming a diet high in raw fruits and vegetables.

Blood Type Diet:

Ingredients:

1. Type O: Lean meats (e.g., beef, lamb, turkey), fish, fruits (e.g., berries, plums, figs), vegetables (e.g., kale, spinach, broccoli), olive oil

2. Type A: Plant-based proteins (e.g., tofu, tempeh, legumes), fruits (e.g., berries, apples, pears), vegetables (e.g., spinach, kale, broccoli), grains (e.g., rice, oats, quinoa)

3. Type B: Lean meats (e.g., lamb, rabbit, venison), fish, dairy (e.g., yogurt, feta cheese), eggs, fruits (e.g., plums, grapes, pineapple), vegetables (e.g., beets, broccoli, sweet potatoes)

4. Type AB: Seafood, tofu, dairy (e.g., yogurt, goat cheese), eggs, fruits (e.g., berries, plums, grapes), vegetables (e.g., spinach, kale, broccoli), grains (e.g., rice, oats, quinoa)

Instructions:

1. Identify your blood type: Determine your blood type (O, A, B, or AB) through blood testing or by using a blood type kit available in some pharmacies.

2. Follow food recommendations for your blood type: Choose foods that are recommended for your blood type according to the Blood Type Diet guidelines.

3. Type O diet: Emphasize lean meats, fish, fruits, and vegetables, while minimizing dairy and grains. Engage in regular physical activity, including vigorous exercise.

4. Type A diet: Focus on plant-based proteins, fruits, vegetables, and whole grains, while limiting animal proteins and dairy. Engage in calming activities like yoga and meditation.

5. Type B diet: Include a variety of lean meats, fish, dairy, and eggs, along with fruits, vegetables, and grains. Engage in moderate physical activity like hiking or swimming.

6. Type AB diet: Incorporate seafood, tofu, dairy, eggs, fruits, vegetables, and grains into your diet. Engage in a balanced mix of calming and moderate physical activities.

7. Pay attention to portion sizes: Be mindful of portion sizes and listen to your body's hunger and fullness cues to prevent overeating.

8. Stay hydrated: Drink plenty of water throughout the day to stay hydrated and support overall health, regardless of your blood type.

9. Monitor how foods affect you: Pay attention to how different foods make you feel and adjust your diet accordingly to support your health and well-being.

10. Consult a healthcare professional: Discuss the Blood Type Diet with a healthcare professional or registered dietitian to ensure it aligns with your individual health needs and goals.

By following these guidelines, you can successfully adhere to the Raw Food Diet or Blood Type Diet, promoting better health and well-being through nutrient-rich foods tailored to your dietary preferences or blood type. Remember to consult with a healthcare professional or registered dietitian for personalized guidance and support, especially if you have specific dietary needs or medical conditions.

Candida Diet:

Ingredients:

1. Non-starchy vegetables (e.g., leafy greens, broccoli, cauliflower, zucchini)

2. Low-sugar fruits (e.g., berries, green apples, citrus fruits)

3. Lean proteins (e.g., chicken, turkey, fish, tofu)

4. Healthy fats (e.g., avocado, olive oil, coconut oil)

5. Fermented foods (e.g., sauerkraut, kimchi, kefir)

6. Herbs and spices (e.g., garlic, ginger, turmeric, cinnamon)

7. Nuts and seeds (e.g., almonds, walnuts, chia seeds, flaxseeds)

8. Non-dairy alternatives (e.g., almond milk, coconut yogurt)

9. Stevia or other natural sweeteners (in moderation)

10.	Herbal teas and water

Instructions:

1. Eliminate sugar and refined carbs: Remove sugar, refined carbohydrates, and high-sugar fruits from your diet, as they can feed candida overgrowth. This includes avoiding sweets, sugary beverages, white bread, pasta, and processed snacks.

2. Focus on non-starchy vegetables: Base your meals around non-starchy vegetables, which are low in sugar and provide fiber and essential nutrients. These include leafy greens, cruciferous vegetables, and other colorful veggies.

3. Choose low-sugar fruits: Enjoy low-sugar fruits such as berries, green apples, and citrus fruits in moderation, as they contain fewer sugars that can exacerbate candida overgrowth.

4. Include lean proteins: Incorporate lean sources of protein like chicken, turkey, fish, and tofu to support muscle health and satiety.

5. Use healthy fats: Opt for healthy fats like avocado, olive oil, and coconut oil to add flavor and healthy calories to your meals.

6. Include fermented foods: Incorporate fermented foods like sauerkraut, kimchi, and kefir into your diet to promote gut health and balance the microbiome.

7. Flavor with herbs and spices: Use herbs and spices like garlic, ginger, turmeric, and cinnamon to add flavor to your meals without relying on sugar or processed condiments.

8. Snack on nuts and seeds: Enjoy nuts and seeds like almonds, walnuts, chia seeds, and flaxseeds as nutrient-rich snacks that provide healthy fats, protein, and fiber.

9. Opt for non-dairy alternatives: Choose non-dairy alternatives like almond milk and coconut yogurt to avoid the lactose found in dairy products, which can exacerbate candida overgrowth.

10. Stay hydrated: Drink plenty of water throughout the day to stay hydrated and support detoxification processes, which can help alleviate candida symptoms.

Specific Carbohydrate Diet (SCD):

Ingredients:

1. Fresh fruits (e.g., bananas, apples, berries)

2. Non-starchy vegetables (e.g., spinach, kale, carrots, zucchini)

3. Lean proteins (e.g., chicken, turkey, fish, eggs)

4. Nuts and seeds (e.g., almonds, pecans, pumpkin seeds, sunflower seeds)

5. Healthy fats (e.g., olive oil, avocado, coconut oil)

6. Homemade bone broth

7. Homemade yogurt (fermented for at least 24 hours)

8. Honey (in moderation)

9. Herbs and spices (e.g., basil, oregano, turmeric, ginger)

10. Water and herbal teas

Instructions:

1. Eliminate specific carbohydrates: Remove complex carbohydrates like grains, starches, and certain sugars from your diet, as they can feed harmful bacteria and worsen digestive symptoms. This includes avoiding wheat, barley, corn, and most processed foods.

2. Emphasize fresh fruits and vegetables: Base your meals around fresh fruits and non-starchy vegetables, which provide essential nutrients and fiber without exacerbating digestive issues.

3. Include lean proteins: Incorporate lean sources of protein like chicken, turkey, fish, and eggs to support muscle health and provide essential amino acids.

4. Snack on nuts and seeds: Enjoy nuts and seeds like almonds, pecans, pumpkin seeds, and sunflower seeds as nutrient-rich snacks that provide healthy fats and protein.

5. Use healthy fats: Opt for healthy fats like olive oil, avocado, and coconut oil to add flavor and satiety to your meals without relying on processed oils or trans fats.

6. Make homemade bone broth: Prepare homemade bone broth using high-quality bones and vegetables to support gut health and provide essential nutrients like collagen and amino acids.

7. Ferment yogurt at home: Make homemade yogurt and ferment it for at least 24 hours to remove lactose and increase beneficial bacteria, which can support digestion and reduce symptoms.

8. Sweeten with honey: Use honey in moderation as a natural sweetener, as it is allowed on the Specific Carbohydrate Diet and provides additional nutrients and antioxidants.

9. Flavor with herbs and spices: Use herbs and spices like basil, oregano, turmeric, and ginger to add flavor to your meals without relying on processed sauces or condiments.

10. Stay hydrated: Drink plenty of water throughout the day to stay hydrated and support overall health, especially when following a restrictive diet like the Specific Carbohydrate Diet.

By following these guidelines, you can successfully adhere to the Candida Diet or Specific Carbohydrate Diet, promoting better digestive health and well-being through balanced nutrition and dietary habits tailored to your individual needs. Remember to consult with a healthcare professional or registered dietitian for personalized guidance and support, especially if you have specific dietary needs or medical conditions.

GAPS Diet:

Ingredients:

1. Homemade bone broth (from organic, pasture-raised animals)

2. Non-starchy vegetables (e.g., broccoli, cauliflower, spinach, kale)

3. Fermented foods (e.g., sauerkraut, kimchi, kefir)

4. Healthy fats (e.g., avocado, coconut oil, olive oil)

5. Wild-caught fish (e.g., salmon, mackerel, sardines)

6. Grass-fed meats (e.g., beef, lamb, poultry)

7. Pastured eggs

8. Nuts and seeds (e.g., almonds, walnuts, flaxseeds, chia seeds)

9. Low-sugar fruits (e.g., berries, green apples, citrus fruits)

10.   Herbal teas and filtered water

Instructions:

1. Eliminate processed foods: Remove processed foods, refined carbohydrates, sugars, and artificial additives from your diet, as they can contribute to gut dysbiosis and inflammation.

2. Start with homemade bone broth: Incorporate homemade bone broth made from organic, pasture-raised animals into your diet to support gut health and provide essential nutrients like collagen and amino acids.

3. Include non-starchy vegetables: Base your meals around non-starchy vegetables like broccoli, cauliflower, spinach, and kale, which provide fiber, vitamins, minerals, and phytonutrients.

4. Incorporate fermented foods: Include fermented foods like sauerkraut, kimchi, and kefir to introduce beneficial probiotics into your gut and support digestive health.

5. Choose healthy fats: Opt for healthy fats like avocado, coconut oil, and olive oil to provide essential fatty acids and support cellular function and inflammation regulation.

6. Include wild-caught fish: Incorporate wild-caught fish like salmon, mackerel, and sardines into your diet as sources of omega-3 fatty acids, which have anti-inflammatory properties.

7. Select grass-fed meats: Choose grass-fed meats like beef, lamb, and poultry over conventionally raised meats to reduce exposure to antibiotics and hormones and increase nutrient content.

8. Include pastured eggs: Incorporate pastured eggs into your diet as a source of protein and essential nutrients like choline and vitamin D.

9. Snack on nuts and seeds: Enjoy nuts and seeds like almonds, walnuts, flaxseeds, and chia seeds as nutrient-rich snacks that provide healthy fats, protein, and fiber.

10. Enjoy low-sugar fruits: Choose low-sugar fruits like berries, green apples, and citrus fruits in moderation to satisfy sweet cravings without spiking blood sugar levels.

Wahls Protocol:

Ingredients:

1. Colorful vegetables (e.g., kale, spinach, beets, carrots, sweet potatoes)

2. Cruciferous vegetables (e.g., broccoli, Brussels sprouts, cauliflower)

3. Berries (e.g., blueberries, strawberries, raspberries)

4. Grass-fed meats (e.g., beef, lamb, bison)

5. Wild-caught fish (e.g., salmon, mackerel, sardines)

6. Organ meats (e.g., liver, heart)

7. Healthy fats (e.g., avocado, coconut oil, olive oil)

8. Fermented foods (e.g., sauerkraut, kimchi, kombucha)

9. Nuts and seeds (e.g., almonds, walnuts, flaxseeds, chia seeds)

10.   Bone broth and collagen peptides

Instructions:

1. Prioritize colorful vegetables: Base your meals around colorful vegetables like kale, spinach, beets, carrots, and sweet potatoes, which provide essential nutrients and antioxidants.

2. Include cruciferous vegetables: Incorporate cruciferous vegetables like broccoli, Brussels sprouts, and cauliflower

into your diet for their anti-inflammatory properties and potential cancer-fighting benefits.

3. Enjoy berries: Include a variety of berries such as blueberries, strawberries, and raspberries in your diet for their antioxidant content and potential neuroprotective effects.

4. Choose grass-fed meats: Opt for grass-fed meats like beef, lamb, and bison over conventionally raised meats to reduce exposure to antibiotics and hormones and increase omega-3 fatty acid content.

5. Include wild-caught fish: Incorporate wild-caught fish like salmon, mackerel, and sardines into your diet as sources of omega-3 fatty acids and protein.

6. Incorporate organ meats: Include organ meats like liver and heart into your diet for their concentrated nutrient content, including vitamins, minerals, and essential amino acids.

7. Use healthy fats: Choose healthy fats like avocado, coconut oil, and olive oil to provide essential fatty acids and support cellular function and inflammation regulation.

8. Include fermented foods: Incorporate fermented foods like sauerkraut, kimchi, and kombucha to introduce beneficial probiotics into your gut and support digestive health.

9. Snack on nuts and seeds: Enjoy nuts and seeds like almonds, walnuts, flaxseeds, and chia seeds as nutrient-rich snacks that provide healthy fats, protein, and fiber.

10.   Include bone broth and collagen peptides: Incorporate bone broth and collagen peptides into your diet to support gut health, joint function, and skin health.

By following these guidelines, you can successfully adhere to the GAPS Diet or Wahls Protocol, promoting better health and well-being through balanced nutrition and dietary habits tailored to support gut health, inflammation regulation, and overall vitality. Remember to consult with a healthcare professional or registered dietitian for personalized guidance and support, especially if you have specific dietary needs or medical conditions.

Pegan Diet:

Ingredients:

1. Plant-based foods: Fruits, vegetables, legumes, nuts, seeds, and whole grains form the foundation of the Pegan diet.

2. Lean proteins: Small portions of sustainably sourced animal proteins such as fish, poultry, and occasionally grass-fed meats are allowed.

3. Healthy fats: Avocado, olive oil, nuts, seeds, and coconut oil are encouraged as sources of healthy fats.

4. Limited dairy: Dairy products are limited or avoided, with emphasis placed on non-dairy alternatives like almond milk or coconut yogurt.

5. Whole grains: Whole grains such as quinoa, brown rice, and oats are included, but in moderate amounts.

6. No processed foods: Highly processed foods, refined sugars, and artificial additives are strictly limited or eliminated.

7. Low glycemic index: Emphasis is placed on choosing foods with a low glycemic index to help stabilize blood sugar levels.

8. Colorful fruits and vegetables: A variety of colorful fruits and vegetables are encouraged to maximize nutrient intake and antioxidant levels.

9. Mindful eating: Attention is given to portion sizes and mindful eating practices to foster a healthy relationship with food.

10. Hydration: Drinking plenty of water throughout the day is essential for overall health and hydration.

Instructions:

1. Fill your plate with vegetables: Aim to make vegetables the main component of your meals, filling at least half of your plate with a variety of colorful veggies.

2. Include plant-based proteins: Incorporate plant-based protein sources such as beans, lentils, tofu, and tempeh into your meals.

3. Choose quality animal proteins: When consuming animal proteins, opt for sustainably sourced options like wild-caught fish, free-range poultry, and grass-fed meats.

4. Prioritize healthy fats: Include sources of healthy fats like avocado, olive oil, nuts, and seeds in your meals to support heart health and satiety.

5. Limit dairy intake: Minimize consumption of dairy products and opt for non-dairy alternatives like almond milk or coconut yogurt when possible.

6. Opt for whole grains: Choose whole grains like quinoa, brown rice, and oats over refined grains to increase fiber intake and stabilize blood sugar levels.

7. Avoid processed foods: Steer clear of highly processed foods, refined sugars, and artificial additives, focusing instead on whole, unprocessed foods.

8. Emphasize low-glycemic foods: Select foods with a low glycemic index to help manage blood sugar levels and reduce the risk of insulin resistance.

9. Eat mindfully: Pay attention to portion sizes and practice mindful eating by slowing down and savoring each bite.

10.   Stay hydrated: Drink plenty of water throughout the day to stay hydrated and support overall health and well-being.

Low-Sodium Diet:

Ingredients:

1. Fresh fruits and vegetables: Choose a variety of fresh fruits and vegetables as the foundation of your meals.

2. Lean proteins: Include lean sources of protein such as poultry, fish, tofu, and legumes in your diet.

3. Whole grains: Opt for whole grains like brown rice, quinoa, and whole wheat bread over refined grains.

4. Herbs and spices: Use herbs, spices, and citrus juices to flavor your meals instead of salt.

5. Low-sodium condiments: Choose low-sodium or sodium-free condiments like mustard, vinegar, and salsa.

6. Unsalted nuts and seeds: Snack on unsalted nuts and seeds for a crunchy and nutritious option.

7. Low-sodium dairy: Select low-sodium or sodium-free dairy products like milk, yogurt, and cheese.

8. Fresh or frozen foods: Prioritize fresh or frozen foods over canned or processed options, which often contain high levels of sodium.

9. Homemade meals: Prepare homemade meals whenever possible to have better control over the sodium content.

10. Water: Drink plenty of water throughout the day to stay hydrated and flush out excess sodium from your body.

Instructions:

1. Read food labels: Check food labels for sodium content and choose products with lower sodium levels.

2. Cook from scratch: Prepare meals at home using fresh ingredients to control the amount of salt added to your food.

3. Flavor with herbs and spices: Use herbs, spices, and citrus juices to add flavor to your meals without relying on salt.

4. Rinse canned foods: If using canned foods, rinse them under water to remove excess sodium before consuming.

5. Limit processed foods: Minimize consumption of processed and packaged foods, which often contain high levels of sodium.

6. Be mindful of condiments: Choose low-sodium or sodium-free condiments and sauces, and use them sparingly.

7. Experiment with alternative seasonings: Try alternative seasonings like garlic powder, onion powder, lemon zest, or vinegar to add flavor to your dishes.

8. Reduce salty snacks: Cut back on salty snacks like chips, pretzels, and salted nuts, opting for unsalted alternatives instead.

9. Choose low-sodium options: When dining out or ordering takeout, opt for dishes labeled as low-sodium or ask for sauces and dressings on the side.

10. Monitor portion sizes: Be mindful of portion sizes, as even low-sodium foods can contribute to high sodium intake if consumed in large amounts.

By following these guidelines, you can successfully adhere to the Pegan Diet or Low-Sodium Diet, promoting better health and well-being through balanced nutrition and mindful dietary habits. Remember to consult with a healthcare professional or registered dietitian for personalized guidance and support, especially if you have specific dietary needs or medical conditions.

Low-Histamine Diet:

Ingredients:

1. Fresh meats: Choose fresh meats such as poultry, fish, and lean cuts of beef or pork.

2. Fresh fruits: Opt for fresh fruits such as apples, pears, berries, and citrus fruits.

3. Fresh vegetables: Include fresh vegetables like leafy greens, broccoli, cauliflower, and carrots.

4. Gluten-free grains: Choose gluten-free grains like rice, quinoa, millet, and buckwheat.

5. Fresh herbs and spices: Flavor your meals with fresh herbs and spices like parsley, basil, ginger, and turmeric.

6. Healthy fats: Incorporate healthy fats like olive oil, avocado oil, coconut oil, and flaxseed oil.

7. Low-histamine dairy alternatives: Opt for low-histamine dairy alternatives such as almond milk or coconut milk.

8. Fresh beverages: Drink fresh water, herbal teas, or fresh juices made from low-histamine fruits and vegetables.

9. Fresh legumes: Include fresh legumes like lentils, chickpeas, and green peas in your diet.

10. Low-histamine sweeteners: Use low-histamine sweeteners such as honey or maple syrup in moderation.

Instructions:

1. Avoid aged and fermented foods: Steer clear of aged and fermented foods such as aged cheeses, cured meats, fermented vegetables, and alcoholic beverages.

2. Minimize processed foods: Limit or avoid processed foods, as they may contain additives and preservatives that can trigger histamine release.

3. Choose fresh over leftovers: Opt for fresh foods over leftovers, as histamine levels increase in foods as they age.

4. Be cautious with high-histamine fruits and vegetables: Some fruits and vegetables, such as tomatoes, spinach, and bananas, may have higher histamine levels when overripe or processed.

5. Monitor histamine levels in meats: Fresh meats are generally lower in histamine compared to processed or aged meats, so choose fresh cuts whenever possible.

6. Consider cooking methods: Grilling, baking, or steaming foods can help reduce histamine levels compared to frying or sautéing.

7. Read labels: Check food labels for ingredients that may contain histamine or trigger histamine release, such as artificial additives or flavorings.

8. Keep a food diary: Keep track of your food intake and any symptoms you experience to identify potential triggers and make adjustments to your diet accordingly.

9. Gradually reintroduce foods: If you eliminate certain foods from your diet, gradually reintroduce them one at a time to monitor your body's response and tolerance.

10.   Consult a healthcare professional: Consider consulting with a healthcare professional or registered dietitian for personalized guidance and support, especially if you have specific dietary needs or medical conditions related to histamine intolerance.

Low-Oxalate Diet:

Ingredients:

1. Low-oxalate fruits: Choose low-oxalate fruits such as apples, pears, berries, and melons.

2. Low-oxalate vegetables: Include low-oxalate vegetables like leafy greens, cucumbers, bell peppers, and cauliflower.

3. Low-oxalate grains: Opt for low-oxalate grains such as white rice, quinoa, oats, and barley.

4. Lean proteins: Incorporate lean protein sources such as poultry, fish, tofu, and eggs.

5. Dairy alternatives: Choose dairy alternatives like almond milk or coconut yogurt if dairy is tolerated.

6. Healthy fats: Include healthy fats like olive oil, avocado oil, nuts, and seeds in moderation.

7. Fresh herbs and spices: Flavor your meals with fresh herbs and spices like basil, oregano, garlic, and ginger.

8. Low-oxalate beverages: Drink low-oxalate beverages such as water, herbal teas, and diluted fruit juices.

9. Low-oxalate legumes: Include low-oxalate legumes like lentils, chickpeas, and green peas in your diet.

10. Low-oxalate sweeteners: Use low-oxalate sweeteners such as honey or maple syrup in moderation.

Instructions:

1. Avoid high-oxalate foods: Steer clear of high-oxalate foods such as spinach, rhubarb, beets, nuts, seeds, and chocolate.

2. Limit high-oxalate beverages: Reduce consumption of high-oxalate beverages such as black tea, green tea, and certain fruit juices like cranberry or grape.

3. Cook vegetables to reduce oxalate content: Boiling, steaming, or blanching vegetables can help reduce their oxalate content compared to eating them raw or sautéed.

4. Soak and cook legumes properly: Soaking and cooking legumes properly can help reduce their oxalate content and improve their digestibility.

5. Consider calcium intake: Adequate calcium intake may help bind oxalates in the gut, so include calcium-rich foods like dairy (if tolerated), fortified non-dairy alternatives, or calcium supplements if needed.

6. Drink plenty of water: Stay well-hydrated by drinking plenty of water throughout the day to help prevent kidney stone formation and support overall health.

7. Keep a food diary: Keep track of your food intake and any symptoms you experience to identify potential triggers and make adjustments to your diet accordingly.

8. Gradually reintroduce foods: If you eliminate certain foods from your diet, gradually reintroduce them one at a time to monitor your body's response and tolerance.

9. Consult a healthcare professional: Consider consulting with a healthcare professional or registered dietitian for personalized guidance and support, especially if you have specific dietary needs or medical conditions related to oxalate sensitivity or kidney stone formation.

Low-Sulfur Diet:

Ingredients:

1. Fresh meats: Choose fresh meats such as poultry, fish, and lean cuts of beef or pork.

2. Fresh fruits: Opt for fresh fruits such as apples, pears, berries, and melons.

3. Fresh vegetables: Include fresh vegetables like leafy greens, carrots, cucumbers, and bell peppers.

4. Low-sulfur grains: Choose low-sulfur grains such as rice, quinoa, millet, and oats.

5. Healthy fats: Incorporate healthy fats like olive oil, avocado, nuts, and seeds.

6. Dairy alternatives: Select dairy alternatives like almond milk or coconut yogurt if dairy is eliminated.

7. Fresh herbs and spices: Flavor your meals with fresh herbs and spices like basil, oregano, garlic, and ginger.

8. Low-sulfur legumes: Include low-sulfur legumes such as lentils, chickpeas, and green peas.

9. Low-sulfur sweeteners: Use low-sulfur sweeteners such as honey or maple syrup in moderation.

10. Water and herbal teas: Drink plenty of water and herbal teas throughout the day to stay hydrated.

Instructions:

1. Identify sulfur-rich foods: Work with a healthcare professional or registered dietitian to identify sulfur-rich foods and sources in your diet.

2. Follow a strict low-sulfur diet: Eliminate high-sulfur foods from your diet for a specified period, typically 2-4 weeks.

3. Keep a food diary: Keep track of your food intake and any symptoms you experience during the low-sulfur diet phase to help identify patterns and trigger foods.

4. Gradually reintroduce foods: After the low-sulfur diet phase, gradually reintroduce eliminated foods one at a time, monitoring your body's response and any symptoms that may occur.

5. Monitor symptoms: Pay close attention to any symptoms or reactions that occur after reintroducing specific foods, noting which foods may trigger symptoms.

6. Consider professional guidance: Consult with a healthcare professional or registered dietitian throughout the process for guidance and support, especially if you have specific dietary needs or medical conditions.

7. Customize your diet: Based on your individual results and symptom management, customize your diet to include foods that are well-tolerated and minimize or avoid foods that trigger symptoms.

8. Maintain a balanced diet: Focus on maintaining a balanced diet that includes a variety of nutrient-rich foods to support overall health and well-being.

9. Continue monitoring: Continue monitoring your symptoms and dietary choices over time to ensure long-term symptom management and overall health.

10. Seek further testing if needed: If symptoms persist or worsen despite dietary changes, consider further testing or evaluation by a healthcare professional to rule out underlying medical conditions or sensitivities.

Fasting Mimicking Diet:

Ingredients:

1. Plant-based foods: Incorporate a variety of plant-based foods such as fruits, vegetables, legumes, nuts, and seeds.

2. Healthy fats: Include sources of healthy fats like olive oil, avocado, nuts, and seeds.

3. Whole grains: Choose whole grains like quinoa, brown rice, oats, and barley.

4. Lean proteins: Opt for lean protein sources such as poultry, fish, tofu, and legumes.

5. Low-calorie soups and broths: Enjoy low-calorie soups and broths made from vegetables and lean proteins.

6. Herbal teas and water: Drink plenty of herbal teas and water throughout the fasting mimicking period to stay hydrated.

7. Nutrient-dense snacks: Include nutrient-dense snacks like raw vegetables, fresh fruits, and small portions of nuts or seeds.

8. Supplements (optional): Consider including supplements recommended by healthcare professionals to ensure nutritional needs are met during the fasting mimicking period.

Instructions:

1. Plan your fasting mimicking period: Determine the duration and frequency of your fasting mimicking diet, typically ranging from 3 to 5 days every 1 to 6 months.

2. Prepare your meals: Plan your meals for the fasting mimicking period, focusing on nutrient-dense, low-calorie foods that provide essential vitamins and minerals.

3. Reduce caloric intake: Limit your caloric intake to around 40-50% of your normal daily caloric intake during the fasting mimicking period.

4. Follow the fasting mimicking protocol: Follow the prescribed fasting mimicking protocol, which typically involves consuming specific meals and snacks designed to mimic the effects of fasting on the body.

5. Monitor your body's response: Pay attention to your body's response during the fasting mimicking period, noting any changes in energy levels, hunger, mood, or other symptoms.

6. Stay hydrated: Drink plenty of water and herbal teas throughout the fasting mimicking period to stay hydrated and support the body's detoxification processes.

7. Break the fast gradually: After completing the fasting mimicking period, gradually reintroduce regular foods into your diet over the course of a few days to avoid digestive discomfort.

8. Monitor long-term effects: Keep track of any long-term benefits or changes in health markers following the fasting mimicking diet, and consult with healthcare professionals as needed.

9. Consider professional guidance: Consult with healthcare professionals or registered dietitians before starting a fasting mimicking diet, especially if you have underlying health conditions or dietary concerns.

10. Customize to your needs: Tailor the fasting mimicking diet to your individual needs and preferences, adjusting the duration, frequency, and specific foods based on your goals and health status.

Intermittent Fasting:

Ingredients: Intermittent fasting does not involve specific ingredients, as it focuses on timing of meals rather than food choices. However, it's important to consume nutrient-dense foods during eating periods to support overall health.

Instructions:

1. Choose an intermittent fasting protocol: Select an intermittent fasting protocol that fits your lifestyle and goals, such as the 16/8 method, 5:2 method, or alternate day fasting.

2. Determine your fasting and eating windows: Establish the duration of your fasting and eating windows based on your chosen intermittent fasting protocol.

3. Plan your meals: Plan balanced meals that include nutrient-dense foods to consume during your eating windows.

4. Stay hydrated: Drink plenty of water during fasting periods to stay hydrated and support overall health.

5. Monitor your body's response: Pay attention to your body's response to intermittent fasting, including changes in hunger, energy levels, mood, and other symptoms.

6. Adjust as needed: Adjust your intermittent fasting protocol as needed based on your individual response and goals.

7. Consider professional guidance: Consult with healthcare professionals or registered dietitians before starting intermittent fasting, especially if you have underlying health conditions or dietary concerns.

8. Be consistent: Stick to your intermittent fasting schedule consistently to maximize potential benefits and adapt to the fasting routine.

9. Listen to your body: Listen to your body's hunger and fullness cues during eating windows, and adjust your meal timing and portion sizes accordingly.

10. Monitor long-term effects: Keep track of any long-term benefits or changes in health markers following intermittent fasting, and consult with healthcare professionals as needed.

Calorie Restriction Diet:

Ingredients:

1. Nutrient-dense foods: Include nutrient-dense foods that provide essential vitamins, minerals, and antioxidants.

2. Lean proteins: Opt for lean protein sources such as poultry, fish, tofu, legumes, and low-fat dairy products.

3. Whole grains: Choose whole grains like brown rice, quinoa, oats, and whole wheat bread to provide sustained energy.

4. Healthy fats: Incorporate healthy fats like olive oil, avocado, nuts, and seeds in moderation to support heart health.

5. Fresh fruits and vegetables: Include a variety of colorful fruits and vegetables to provide fiber and essential nutrients.

6. Low-calorie snacks: Enjoy low-calorie snacks such as raw vegetables, fresh fruits, and air-popped popcorn to satisfy hunger between meals.

7. Herbal teas and water: Drink plenty of herbal teas and water throughout the day to stay hydrated and support digestion.

8. Supplements (optional): Consider including supplements recommended by healthcare professionals to ensure nutritional needs are met while reducing calorie intake.

Instructions:

1. Determine your calorie goal: Calculate your daily calorie goal based on your individual needs, goals, and activity level.

2. Plan your meals: Plan balanced meals that include a variety of nutrient-dense foods while staying within your calorie limit.

3. Monitor portion sizes: Pay attention to portion sizes to ensure you're consuming the appropriate amount of calories for your goals.

4. Track your intake: Keep track of your calorie intake using a food diary or tracking app to stay accountable and monitor progress.

5. Focus on nutrient density: Prioritize nutrient-dense foods that provide essential vitamins, minerals, and antioxidants to support overall health.

6. Eat mindfully: Practice mindful eating by slowing down, savoring each bite, and paying attention to hunger and fullness cues.

7. Include protein at each meal: Incorporate lean protein sources at each meal to support muscle health and promote satiety.

8. Choose low-calorie snacks: Opt for low-calorie snacks like raw vegetables, fresh fruits, and air-popped popcorn to satisfy hunger between meals without exceeding your calorie limit.

9. Stay hydrated: Drink plenty of water and herbal teas throughout the day to stay hydrated and support digestion.

10. Monitor progress: Regularly assess your progress towards your calorie restriction goals and make adjustments as needed to ensure sustainable and healthy weight management.

MIND Diet:

Ingredients:

1. Leafy greens: Include leafy greens such as spinach, kale, and Swiss chard as a staple in your diet.

2. Other vegetables: Incorporate a variety of other vegetables like broccoli, carrots, bell peppers, and tomatoes.

3. Berries: Enjoy a variety of berries such as blueberries, strawberries, raspberries, and blackberries as a rich source of antioxidants.

4. Whole grains: Choose whole grains like oats, brown rice, quinoa, and whole wheat bread to provide fiber and essential nutrients.

5. Fish: Include fatty fish such as salmon, mackerel, tuna, and sardines as a source of omega-3 fatty acids.

6. Poultry: Opt for poultry like chicken or turkey as a lean protein source.

7. Nuts: Incorporate nuts such as almonds, walnuts, and cashews for healthy fats and protein.

8. Olive oil: Use olive oil as your primary source of fat for cooking and dressing salads.

9. Beans: Include beans such as lentils, chickpeas, black beans, and kidney beans for fiber and protein.

10.   Wine (optional): Enjoy red wine in moderation, if desired, as part of the MIND diet's recommendations.

Instructions:

1. Prioritize plant-based foods: Base your meals around plant-based foods such as leafy greens, vegetables, fruits, and whole grains.

2. Include berries regularly: Aim to include berries in your diet several times a week, as they are rich in antioxidants and linked to brain health.

3. Choose healthy fats: Opt for sources of healthy fats like olive oil, nuts, and fatty fish to support brain function and heart health.

4. Limit red meat and processed foods: Reduce consumption of red meat and processed foods, as they are associated with negative health outcomes.

5. Eat fish at least twice a week: Include fatty fish in your diet at least twice a week to benefit from omega-3 fatty acids.

6. Include poultry and beans: Incorporate poultry and beans regularly as sources of lean protein and fiber.

7. Enjoy nuts daily: Include a handful of nuts in your daily diet for their beneficial nutrients and satiating effects.

8. Cook with olive oil: Use olive oil as your primary cooking oil and salad dressing to add flavor and promote heart health.

9. Limit sweets and pastries: Reduce consumption of sweets, pastries, and high-fat dairy products, as they are not part of the MIND diet's recommendations.

10. Moderate wine intake: If desired, enjoy red wine in moderation, as it is associated with certain health benefits when consumed in moderation. However, avoid excessive alcohol intake, as it can have negative effects on health.

By following these guidelines, you can successfully adhere to the Calorie Restriction Diet or MIND Diet, promoting better health and well-being through balanced nutrition and mindful dietary habits. Remember to consult with a healthcare professional or registered dietitian for personalized guidance and support, especially if you have specific dietary needs or medical conditions.

TLC Diet (Therapeutic Lifestyle Changes Diet):

Ingredients:

1. Fruits: Include a variety of fresh fruits such as berries, apples, oranges, and bananas.

2. Vegetables: Incorporate a wide range of vegetables like leafy greens, broccoli, carrots, tomatoes, and bell peppers.

3. Whole grains: Choose whole grains like oats, barley, quinoa, brown rice, and whole wheat bread.

4. Lean proteins: Opt for lean protein sources such as poultry without skin, fish, tofu, legumes, and egg whites.

5. Low-fat dairy: Include low-fat dairy products like skim milk, yogurt, and cheese.

6. Healthy fats: Incorporate healthy fats from sources like olive oil, avocado, nuts, and seeds.

7. Beans and legumes: Include beans and legumes such as lentils, chickpeas, black beans, and kidney beans for protein and fiber.

8. Fish: Incorporate fatty fish like salmon, mackerel, and trout at least twice a week for omega-3 fatty acids.

9. Herbs and spices: Flavor your meals with herbs and spices like garlic, ginger, turmeric, basil, and oregano instead of salt.

10. Water: Drink plenty of water throughout the day to stay hydrated and support overall health.

Instructions:

1. Reduce saturated fat intake: Limit saturated fat intake to less than 7% of total calories by choosing lean protein sources, low-fat dairy, and healthy fats.

2. Limit dietary cholesterol: Aim for less than 200 milligrams of cholesterol per day by choosing lean protein sources and limiting high-cholesterol foods.

3. Increase fiber intake: Include plenty of fiber-rich foods like fruits, vegetables, whole grains, beans, and legumes to promote heart health and digestion.

4. Choose low-sodium options: Opt for low-sodium foods and seasonings to reduce salt intake and support blood pressure management.

5. Limit sugar and refined carbohydrates: Reduce consumption of sugary foods and refined carbohydrates, opting instead for whole grains and natural sweeteners in moderation.

6. Monitor portion sizes: Pay attention to portion sizes to avoid overeating and maintain calorie balance for weight management.

7. Be physically active: Incorporate regular physical activity into your daily routine to support heart health and overall well-being.

8. Monitor progress: Regularly monitor your progress in reducing cholesterol levels and improving heart health, and adjust your diet and lifestyle as needed.

9. Seek professional guidance: Consult with a healthcare professional or registered dietitian for personalized guidance

and support, especially if you have specific dietary needs or medical conditions related to heart health.

10.   Stay consistent: Stick to the TLC diet guidelines consistently to achieve long-term improvements in cholesterol levels and heart health.

Nutritarian Diet:

Ingredients:

1. Vegetables: Base your meals around a variety of colorful vegetables such as leafy greens, cruciferous vegetables, peppers, tomatoes, and carrots.

2. Fruits: Include a variety of fresh fruits such as berries, apples, oranges, grapes, and melons.

3. Beans and legumes: Incorporate beans and legumes such as lentils, chickpeas, black beans, and edamame for protein and fiber.

4. Nuts and seeds: Enjoy nuts and seeds such as almonds, walnuts, flaxseeds, chia seeds, and hemp seeds for healthy fats and protein.

5. Whole grains: Choose whole grains like quinoa, brown rice, oats, barley, and whole wheat pasta for fiber and nutrients.

6. Healthy fats: Include sources of healthy fats like avocado, olive oil, coconut oil, and fatty fish such as salmon and sardines.

7. Herbs and spices: Flavor your meals with herbs and spices like garlic, ginger, turmeric, basil, and cinnamon instead of salt and sugar.

8. Mushrooms: Incorporate mushrooms such as shiitake, portobello, and maitake for their immune-boosting and anti-inflammatory properties.

9. Onions and garlic: Include onions, shallots, leeks, and garlic for their flavor and health-promoting properties.

10. Nutrient-rich beverages: Drink nutrient-rich beverages such as green tea, herbal teas, and water infused with lemon or cucumber for hydration and antioxidants.

Instructions:

1. Eat predominantly plant-based: Base your diet on whole, nutrient-rich plant foods like vegetables, fruits, beans, legumes, nuts, seeds, and whole grains.

2. Maximize nutrient density: Focus on foods that are high in nutrients and low in calories, such as leafy greens, berries, and cruciferous vegetables.

3. Limit processed foods: Minimize consumption of processed and refined foods, including sugary snacks, white bread, and packaged snacks.

4. Avoid added sugars and refined carbohydrates: Limit intake of added sugars and refined carbohydrates, opting instead for whole fruits and whole grains.

5. Include sources of healthy fats: Incorporate sources of healthy fats like nuts, seeds, avocado, and fatty fish to support brain health and overall well-being.

6. Prioritize fiber-rich foods: Choose fiber-rich foods like beans, legumes, whole grains, fruits, and vegetables to support digestion and maintain satiety.

7. Focus on variety: Include a wide variety of plant foods in your diet to ensure you're getting a range of nutrients and phytochemicals.

8. Stay hydrated: Drink plenty of water throughout the day to stay hydrated and support overall health and well-being.

9. Be mindful of portion sizes: Pay attention to portion sizes to avoid overeating, even with nutrient-dense foods.

10. Listen to your body: Pay attention to hunger and fullness cues, and eat mindfully to nourish your body and promote satisfaction.

By following these guidelines, you can successfully adhere to the TLC Diet or Nutritarian Diet, promoting better health and well-being through balanced nutrition and mindful dietary habits. Remember to consult with a healthcare professional or registered dietitian for personalized guidance and support, especially if you have specific dietary needs or medical conditions.

Macro Diet:

Ingredients:

1. Protein sources: Include lean protein sources such as chicken breast, turkey, tofu, tempeh, fish, eggs, and low-fat dairy products.

2. Carbohydrate sources: Choose complex carbohydrates like whole grains (brown rice, quinoa, oats), legumes (beans, lentils), starchy vegetables (sweet potatoes, squash), and fruits.

3. Healthy fats: Incorporate sources of healthy fats such as avocados, nuts, seeds, olive oil, coconut oil, and fatty fish (salmon, mackerel, sardines).

4. Vegetables: Include a variety of non-starchy vegetables like leafy greens, broccoli, cauliflower, bell peppers, cucumbers, and tomatoes.

5. Herbs and spices: Flavor your meals with herbs and spices like garlic, ginger, turmeric, basil, cilantro, and rosemary.

6. Condiments and sauces: Use condiments and sauces sparingly, opting for low-calorie options or making your own with healthy ingredients.

7. Beverages: Drink plenty of water throughout the day, and opt for unsweetened beverages such as herbal teas, black coffee, and sparkling water.

Instructions:

1. Calculate your macros: Determine your daily macronutrient goals based on your individual needs, goals, and activity level (protein, carbohydrates, fats).

2. Plan your meals: Plan balanced meals that align with your macro goals, ensuring each meal includes a source of protein, carbohydrates, and healthy fats.

3. Track your macros: Use a food diary or tracking app to monitor your daily intake of protein, carbohydrates, and fats, adjusting portion sizes and food choices as needed to meet your goals.

4. Prioritize protein: Aim to include a source of protein in each meal to support muscle growth and repair, as well as feelings of fullness and satiety.

5. Choose complex carbohydrates: Opt for complex carbohydrates that provide sustained energy and fiber,

helping to regulate blood sugar levels and promote digestive health.

6. Include healthy fats: Incorporate sources of healthy fats to support hormone production, brain function, and overall health, while moderating portion sizes to manage calorie intake.

7. Eat plenty of vegetables: Fill up on non-starchy vegetables to add volume and nutrients to your meals while keeping calorie counts low.

8. Be mindful of portion sizes: Pay attention to portion sizes to ensure you're consuming the appropriate amount of each macronutrient to meet your goals.

9. Adjust as needed: Monitor your progress and adjust your macro ratios and portion sizes as needed to achieve your desired outcomes.

10.   Seek professional guidance: Consult with a registered dietitian or nutritionist for personalized guidance and support, especially if you have specific dietary needs or medical conditions.

Elimination Diet:

Ingredients:

1. Lean proteins: Choose lean sources of protein such as poultry, fish, tofu, and eggs.

2. Non-allergenic grains: Opt for non-allergenic grains such as rice, quinoa, millet, and oats.

3. Fresh fruits: Include fresh fruits such as apples, pears, berries, and melons.

4. Fresh vegetables: Choose fresh vegetables like leafy greens, carrots, cucumbers, and bell peppers.

5. Healthy fats: Incorporate healthy fats like olive oil, avocado, nuts, and seeds.

6. Dairy alternatives: Select dairy alternatives like almond milk or coconut yogurt if dairy is eliminated.

7. Fresh herbs and spices: Flavor your meals with fresh herbs and spices like basil, oregano, garlic, and ginger.

8. Low-allergen legumes: Include low-allergen legumes such as lentils, chickpeas, and green peas.

9. Low-allergen sweeteners: Use low-allergen sweeteners such as honey or maple syrup in moderation.

10. Water and herbal teas: Drink plenty of water and herbal teas throughout the day to stay hydrated.

Instructions:

1. Identify potential trigger foods: Work with a healthcare professional or registered dietitian to identify potential trigger foods based on your symptoms and health history.

2. Follow a strict elimination phase: Eliminate all potential trigger foods from your diet for a specified period, typically 2-4 weeks.

3. Keep a food diary: Keep track of your food intake and any symptoms you experience during the elimination phase to help identify patterns and trigger foods.

4. Gradually reintroduce foods: After the elimination phase, gradually reintroduce eliminated foods one at a time, monitoring your body's response and any symptoms that may occur.

5. Monitor symptoms: Pay close attention to any symptoms or reactions that occur after reintroducing specific foods, noting which foods may trigger symptoms.

6. Consider professional guidance: Consult with a healthcare professional or registered dietitian throughout the process for guidance and support, especially if you have specific dietary needs or medical conditions.

7. Customize your diet: Based on your individual results and symptom management, customize your diet to include foods

that are well-tolerated and minimize or avoid foods that trigger symptoms.

8. Maintain a balanced diet: Focus on maintaining a balanced diet that includes a variety of nutrient-rich foods to support overall health and well-being.

9. Continue monitoring: Continue monitoring your symptoms and dietary choices over time to ensure long-term symptom management and overall health.

10.   Seek further testing if needed: If symptoms persist or worsen despite dietary changes, consider further testing or evaluation by a healthcare professional to rule out underlying medical conditions or food sensitivities.

THE END

Printed in Great Britain
by Amazon

45636196R00059